W9-DFE-220

FEVER

FEVER

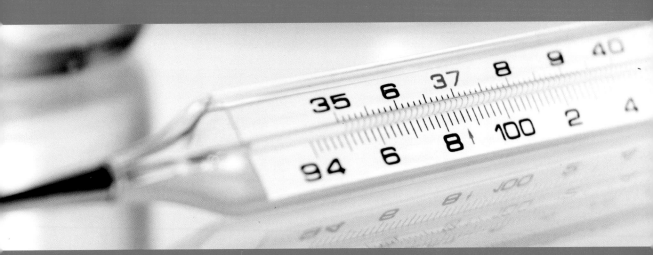

Camilla Calamandrei

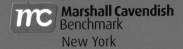

Marshall Cavendish
Benchmark
New York

With thanks to Adam J. Adler, Ph.D., Associate Professor, Center for Immunotherapy of Cancer and Infectious Diseases and Department of Immunology, University of Connecticut Health Center, for his expert review of the manuscript.

Marshall Cavendish Benchmark
99 White Plains Road
Tarrytown, New York 10591-5502
www.marshallcavendish.us

Text copyright © 2009 by Marshall Cavendish Corporation

All rights reserved. No part of this book may be reproduced or utilized in any form or by any means electronic or mechanical including photocopying, recording, or by any information storage and retrieval system, without permission from the copyright holders.

This book is not intended for use as a substitute for advice, consultation, or treatment by a licensed medical practitioner. The reader is advised that no action of a medical nature should be taken without consultation with a licensed medical practitioner, including action that may seem to be indicated by the contents of this work, since individual circumstances vary and medical standards, knowledge, and practices change with time. The publisher, author, and medical consultants disclaim all liability and cannot be held responsible for any problems that may arise from use of this book.

Library of Congress Cataloging-in-Publication Data

Calamandrei, Camilla.
Fever / by Camilla Calamandrei.
p. cm. — (Health alert)
Summary: "Provides comprehensive information on the causes, treatment, and history of fever"—Provided by publisher.
Includes index.
ISBN 978-0-7614-2915-9
1. Fever—Juvenile literature. I. Title. II. Series.
RB129.C24 2009
616'.047—dc22

2007026002

Photo Research by Candlepants Incorporated
Cover: Elynn Cohen
The photographs in this book are used by permission and through the courtesy of:
Photo Researchers Inc.: Gusto, 3; LSHTM, 5; AJPhoto, 9; Grapes & Michaud, 12; Dr. Linda Stannard, UCT, 20; Ian Boddy, 22; James Cavallini, 25; Jim Dowdalls, 27; Bouree (Dr), 29; Andy Crump, TDR, WHO, 31; Eye of Science, 33; VEM, 37; Science Source, 39; Alix, 44; Samuel Ashfield, 45; Andrew Lambert Photography, 46; Mark Clarke, 51; Lea Paterson, 52. *Corbis*: Mascarucci, 11; Ragnar Schmuck/zefa, 12; Kim Ludbrook /epa, 14; Creasource, 16; Visuals Unlimited, 26; Orlando Barría/EFE, 35; Mario Lopez/epa, 36; David Lees, 40; Krista Kennell/ZUMA, 53; Randy Faris, 55; Sandra Seckinger/zefa, 56; Ariel Skelley, 58. *Alamy Images*: Picture Partners , 19. *The Image Works*: Science Museum/SSPL, 41; SSPL, 43; Mary Evans Picture Library, 48.

Editor: Joy Bean
Publisher: Michelle Bisson
Art Director: Anahid Hamparian

Printed in Malaysia
6 5 4 3 2 1

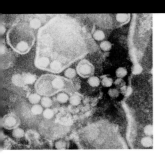

CONTENTS

1

WHAT IS IT LIKE TO HAVE A FEVER?

It was late in the afternoon on a cold winter day but Rhonda was running around her house in a T-shirt and shorts. Her mother and father were each wearing big sweaters and her little brother had flannel pajamas on. At first, Rhonda's mother just thought that Rhonda was being goofy, but Rhonda was comfortable in her lightweight clothes.

By dinnertime, Rhonda felt very tired. She did not feel like eating, she had a headache, and was even shivering. Her dad felt her forehead and noticed that it felt very warm. Using a thermometer, he took Rhonda's temperature. Sure enough, it was 102 degrees Fahrenheit (38.9 degrees Celsius). A normal body temperature for Rhonda, or anyone, would be somewhere around 98.6 °F (37 °C). When a person's body temperature is higher than normal, the person has a **fever**. A fever can be a **symptom**, or sign, of a number of **illnesses**. When someone gets a fever, he or she can feel hot and then cold and then hot again. He or she may start sweating a lot, yet may be shivering.

Rhonda was upset to hear she had a fever because she was afraid that it meant she had to go to the doctor right away. Luckily, her father and mother had a lot of experience dealing with children with fevers. Rhonda's parents knew what to do because Rhonda and her brother had both had fevers before. One time, it turned out they each had **chicken pox**, which is an illness with lots of itchy red spots. Another time, each of them had fevers before they got the **flu**, which is a very common illness that starts out with symptoms like a common head cold. Rhonda and her brother had also gotten fevers when they caught colds. So this time, their parents assumed that Rhonda's fever meant that she was coming down with a cold. Since they did not think that the fever was very high, they decided to wait and see how Rhonda felt the next morning.

Rhonda's parents gave her a big glass of water and then tucked her into bed so that she could rest. However, when her brother came close to kiss her goodnight, Rhonda's parents told him to stay back until Rhonda was feeling better. They were afraid that she was coming down with a cold, which is **contagious**. This means that she could pass her illness on to her brother. The period of time when someone is just beginning to get sick is when they are most likely to be contagious. So, since people tend to get a fever at the beginning of an illness, they are most likely to pass the illness to others while they have the fever. Doctors recommend that children stay home from school, or away from other children, while they have a fever.

The next morning Rhonda woke up feeling worse, but her fever was gone. Instead, she had a sore throat, her nose was running, and she felt achy all over her body. Her parents were sorry that she felt sick, but they were also relieved. These new symptoms, plus the fact that the fever had passed, told them that Rhonda probably had a simple, common cold. They had also spoken to some of their neighbors and heard that a number of kids from Rhonda's class had bad colds. It was most likely that she had caught it from them.

If Rhonda's fever had gotten much higher, or had lasted for more than a day or two, her parents would have taken her to see the doctor. Also, if she had gotten a rash or some other symptom, the doctor would have wanted to see her in person to **diagnose**, or identify, what kind of illness she was getting. Because fevers are associated with so many different kinds of illnesses, it is important to stay on the lookout for additional signs and symptoms that will help a doctor to diagnose sickness.

Rhonda stayed home from school for one day, just to make sure that her fever was not coming back. She rested and drank a lot of fluids. Then, the next day, she went back to school, with a packet of tissues in her backpack for her runny nose. A week later, she was feeling 100 percent better and barely remembered that she had had a fever.

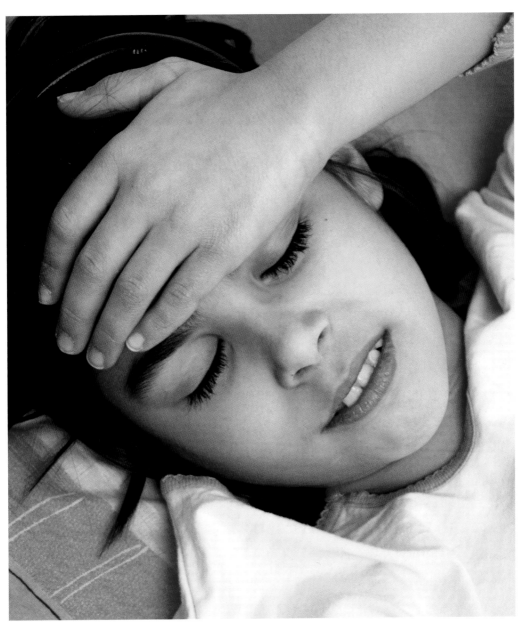

When a person has a fever they may feel achy and tired.

2

WHAT IS A FEVER?

The normal body temperature of an average healthy person is around 98.6 °F (37 °C). When a person's body temperature is more than two or three degrees above that, he or she has a fever, which is also known as **pyrexia.** Small changes in body temperature are very normal and happen every day. Each person's body temperature usually changes by one or two degrees (above and below 98.6 °F) at different times of the day. Most often a person's body temperature will be below average in the early morning hours after the body has rested. That same person's body temperature will usually be higher later in the day after that person has been eating and moving around.

In general, a temperature of 99 to 103 °F (37.2 to 39.4 °C) is considered a mild to moderate fever that is not too serious. Anything above that is considered a more serious fever. A temperature of 108 °F (42.2 °C), would be very unusual and quite dangerous. A fever of 108 °F (42.2° C) or higher can lead

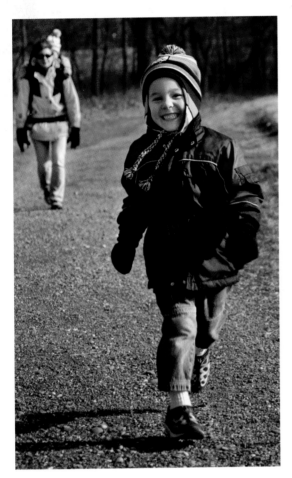

Even when a person is healthy, their body temperature will usually go up a little during the day—especially after they eat or run around.

to convulsions, or violent shaking of muscles, and sometimes even death. Someone with such a high fever should go to a hospital emergency room immediately.

GETTING SICK

Fever is a symptom of an illness, rather than an illness itself. Usually people get a fever when they are sick with an illness like the flu, chicken pox, a cold, or if a wound is infected. Illnesses and **infections** are caused by foreign, or outsider, objects that make their way into the body. These foreign entities that cause illness are called **pathogens**, or **germs**—microorganisms that can infect healthy cells and cause many types of illness. **Viruses** and **bacteria** are kinds of pathogens. They are microorganisms that can infect healthy cells and cause many types of illness.

Pathogens can enter the human body in different ways.

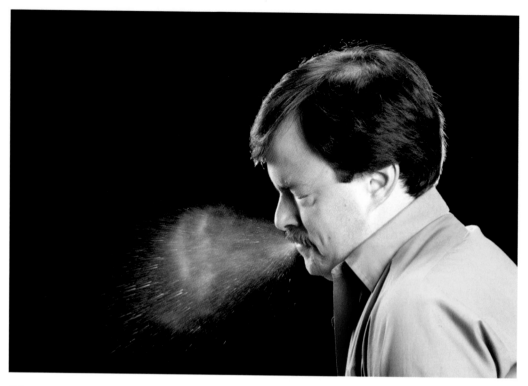

When a person sneezes, germs can spread a great distance.

Some viruses, for example, travel through the air. If someone has a cold or the flu and sneezes, the germs leave the body and are projected into the air. The germs may land on another person's face or in the nose or mouth, spreading the sickness. However, it is more common to catch a cold or flu by your touching something that a sick person has touched and then touching your own face, nose, mouth, or eyes.

Other viruses enter the human body through the bite of an animal or insect. Malaria is an illness that people get when they are bitten by a mosquito infected with the bacteria that causes malaria. Some types of bacteria also enter the body through the bite of an animal or insect. Lyme disease is a bacterial infection caused by the bite of an infected tick.

Sometimes when an animal—such as a mosquito or tick—carries a disease, that animal may not get sick themselves. In that case, the animal or insect is considered an **asymptomatic carrier**, meaning the carrier has no symptoms. People can also be asymptomatic carriers of disease. Once in a while, people can be carrying a contagious disease and not know it. Because they do not know they are sick, they can be exposing many people to the illness and potentially making a lot of people sick.

Another way that germs can enter the body is through fluids, including liquids such as water, blood, and **saliva**, or spit. If there are pathogens in someone's drinking water, for example, he or she can become sick after drinking it. This happens mostly in countries where the people do not have access to clean water. In some countries, people have to bathe in or drink from the same rivers or lakes used for their farm animals, or for washing laundry and other dirty things. In parts of Asia, India, and Africa, unsafe water causes approximately three million deaths a year. Many of the people who die are children, but even adults get sick regularly from dirty water.

People can also become infected with an illness when they

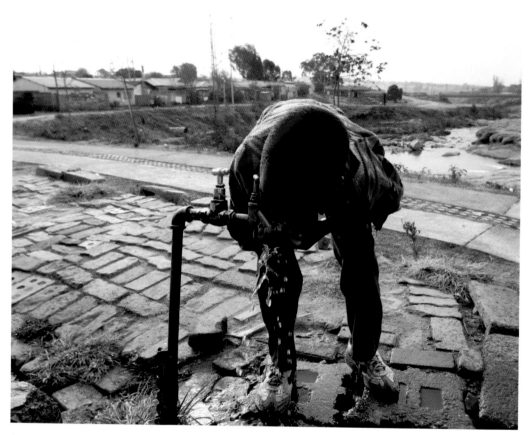

A young boy drinks water from a tap in South Africa.

are exposed to the blood or saliva of another person who is ill. If someone has a cut, or open wound, and he or she touches infected blood from another person, the pathogens can travel from the infected blood into the open cut. This is why dentists, doctors, and emergency workers wear gloves when they are examining patients. If the doctor or dentist had even a small cut on his or her hand, he or she could become infected from

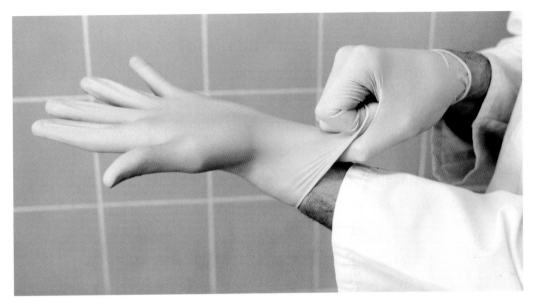

Sometimes doctors wear disposable gloves when they examine a patient. They need to throw out the used gloves and wash their hands before examining the next patient, to make sure they do not spread germs.

the saliva or blood of a patient who was carrying an illness. This is also why people wear bandages. If a wound is covered, it is more likely to be protected from any germs that might be looking for a new place to infect.

INCUBATION

When an infection enters the human body, the bacteria or virus will begin to multiply. During this period, a person may not notice any symptoms at all. This time is called the incubation period for an illness. The incubation period of an illness can last anywhere from a few hours to a few days or weeks depending on the type of illness. During the incubation period, a person may not realize that he or she is sick, and can expose other people to the illness without realizing it. Chicken pox is a good example of an illness that is highly contagious. This is partly because the incubation period is about two weeks long. During that entire period, an infected child can be passing the illness to other children because no one knows yet that the child has chicken pox.

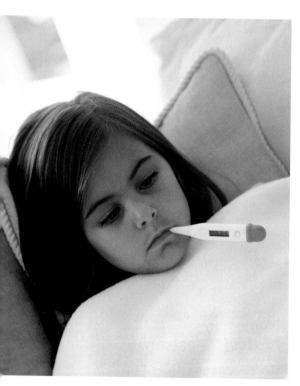

A person may feel cold and shiver when their body temperature is above normal and they have a fever.

THE BODY FIGHTS BACK

Since pathogens can enter the body in so many ways, it is good that the human body has an **immune system** that protects the body from infections and illness. Fever is one of the ways that the immune system fights off pathogens. When a virus or bacteria enters the human body, the body reacts by producing **pyrogens**. Pyrogens are chemicals produced in the body that trick the brain into thinking that the body is cooler than it is. They travel in the blood to the **hypothalamus—**

the part of the brain that keeps the body at the right temperature. As a result, the brain tries to warm the body. This is also why a person who is getting a fever will have the chills, or start shivering. Physical shaking, or shivering, is actually one way the body warms itself up.

When the body stops shivering, the patient will be overheated and feverish but might not feel very hot. This is because the pyrogens are fooling the body into thinking it is a different temperature than it really is. When people are sick they may feel cold when their body is hot, or warm when their body is cold. It can be very confusing! When the pyrogens no longer send the signal to increase the body temperature, the body will try to go back to a normal temperature. During this time, the patient with a fever will feel hot and the body will begin releasing sweat to cool the patient and lower the body temperature. The cycle of getting cold and hot can vary depending on the type of illness a person has. Some illnesses involve a short fever in which people have a fever for a few hours and then it passes. Other types of illness involve fevers that will come and go a number of times.

Although shivering and sweating can be very uncomfortable, the fever itself is actually helping the immune system fight infection in two ways. The first way that an elevated body temperature fights infection is by increasing the movement and multiplication of white blood cells, also called **leukocytes**. The human body has different kinds of white blood cells to fight

Additional Causes of Fever

Although most people will get fevers when they have an infection of some kind, there are some situations in which people with other illnesses or under other kinds of stress may develop fevers. An infant can develop a fever when it is very warm outside and he or she is overdressed. This happens because young babies cannot regulate the temperature of their bodies very well. Babies and children can also get fevers after getting vaccination shots because the body is attacking the small amount of pathogens in the vaccine. (Although a child may get a fever, usually the vaccine will not make the child sick.)

Adults can get fevers as a reaction to a medicine, a blood transfusion, when they have exercised strenuously, or for women, at certain stages in their menstrual cycle. People with cancer may experience fevers as side effects of various treatments. Tumor cells produce substances that can cause fever as well.

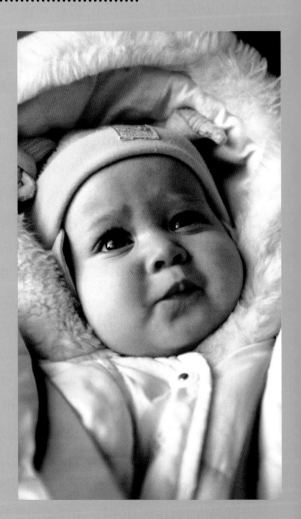

different kinds of germs. Some attack germs by surrounding them and destroying them. Others produce antibodies that keep the germs from growing. In both cases, a fever will get the white blood cells moving and doing their job to combat germs and other pathogens.

The second way an elevated body temperature fights infection is to create an environment in the body that makes it hard for a virus or bacteria to thrive and multiply. Some viruses and bacteria can only live in small ranges of temperatures, so the heat from a fever can actually help kill them off.

COMMON ILLNESSES THAT BEGIN WITH A FEVER

Fever is a symptom that is associated with the beginning of many different kinds of illnesses. Some very common illnesses that have fever as an early symptom are common colds, ear infections, the flu, gastrointestinal infections (which affect your stomach and other digestive organs), strep throat, chicken pox, mononucleosis, urinary tract infections, Coxsackie virus infection, and Lyme disease.

THE COMMON COLD
The common cold is a viral infection of the **upper respiratory tract**, which is made up of the nose and throat. The common cold is very contagious, and travels easily from person to

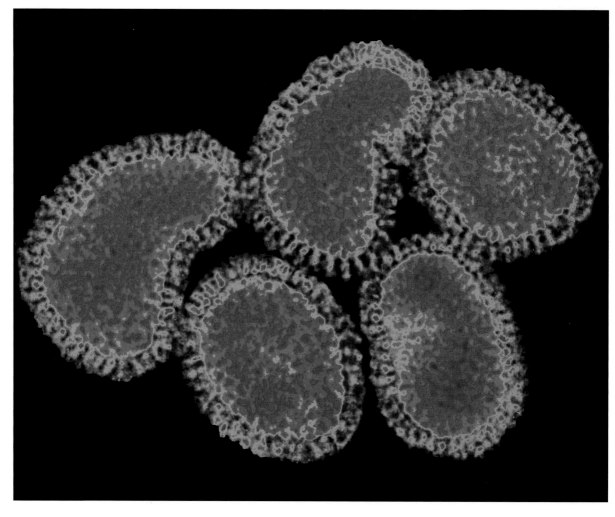

The influenza virus can cause fever, aching muscles, and a sore throat.

person. Some people get mild fevers when they have a cold, and others will not get a fever at all. Because it is caused by a virus, there is no medicine that can cure the common cold. Most people just let the illness run its course, and take medication that helps treat the symptoms.

EAR INFECTIONS

Ear infections occur when germs get trapped in the middle ear. Some children will get mild to moderate fevers when they have an ear infection. Others may get higher fevers if the infection gets quite bad. Most ear infections are treated with antibiotics.

GASTROINTESTINAL INFECTION

Diarrhea (also known as GI or gastrointestinal infection) can be caused by viruses, bacteria, or **parasites**. Children with GI infections will have diarrhea but may also vomit or have a fever and other symptoms. Doctors recommend that patients with GI infections rest and drink a lot of fluids, because diarrhea takes water out of the body. It is very important that the patient drinks enough to replace that water.

STREP THROAT

Strep throat is a highly contagious, bacterial infection that is common in children and teenagers. The primary symptom of strep throat is a sore throat. But not all sore throats are caused by strep bacteria. When someone has a runny nose, and other coldlike symptoms along with a sore throat, it is likely that he or she does not have strep throat. If, however, someone has a sore throat, difficulty swallowing, headaches, pain in the lower stomach, and fever—but no runny nose or cough—he or she may have strep throat. Strep throat is easily diagnosed by a doctor and can be treated with antibiotics.

CHICKEN POX

Chicken pox is caused by a viral infection. It is a common illness in children under twelve years of age, but people can get chicken pox at any age. Some children may feel sick for a few days before coming down with the itchy rash that is chicken pox. Many may also have a low fever. The incubation period for chicken pox is a very long two weeks. This may be part of why it seems to spread so quickly. Many children carrying the illness do not know they are sick during the incubation period and can be passing it to others during those weeks.

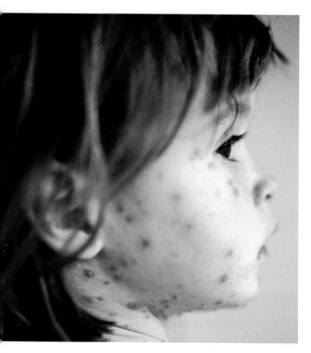

Chicken pox is a common illness for young children.

When a child gets chicken pox, a parent can help the child feel more comfortable by having the child take cool baths every few hours, applying cool wet compresses, or putting calamine lotion on itchy areas. (There is one kind of antiviral medicine that can be used for people with chicken pox, but it is very strong and is not often recommended for children.) If a child scratches the chicken pox blisters, they can become infected. In that case, the doctor may need to prescribe antibiotics.

MONONUCLEOSIS

Mononucleosis, which is commonly called mono, is caused by a widespread virus called Epstein-Barr. Teenagers and young adults who are infected get flulike symptoms, including a fever that can last for a few weeks. The early signs of mono are easily mistaken for the flu. They include fever, sore throat, swollen **lymph nodes** (in the neck, underarms, and groin), exhaustion, and weakness. There is no cure for mono, but medication can be given to help ease the symptoms.

URINARY TRACT INFECTIONS

The urinary tract is the system that removes liquid waste from the body. It includes the kidneys, ureters, bladder, and urethra. Most urinary tract infections are caused by bacterial infection in the urethra or bladder. Sometimes the only sign of a urinary tract infection will be a fever. In other cases, the person will experience pain when urinating. Medication is usually given to get rid of the infection.

COXSACKIE VIRUS

Hand, foot, and mouth disease is caused by the Coxsackie virus. Some children will have no symptoms when they get hand, foot, and mouth disease. Others will have a moderately high fever of 101 to 103 °F (38.3 to 39.4 °C). They may also feel aches in various muscles and have a headache, mild sore throat, or nausea. In many children the fever will disappear after two or three days. In some, however, the fever may last only one day, but may return in two or three days for several more days. There is no medicine to cure the Coxsackie virus. Doctors may suggest a painkiller, such as acetaminophen, to make a child more comfortable.

SERIOUS ILLNESSES THAT BEGIN WITH A FEVER

Some serious illnesses that begin with a fever and can be found around the world are hepatitis, pneumonia, tuberculosis, meningitis, and Q fever. These are illnesses that must be diagnosed and treated by doctors.

HEPATITIS

Hepatitis covers a group of diseases that affect the liver. There are three types of hepatitis: A, B, and C. Hepatitis B can be transmitted from one person to another, and a virus is often the cause. Drinking large amounts of alcohol over many years or exposure to other toxins can also cause hepatitis B. Mild fever can be an early symptom, along with fatigue, loss of appetite, and vomiting. A person with hepatitis B might also feel pain underneath the rib cage near the liver. Hepatitis B can be very dangerous because it can cause long-term liver damage and increase a person's risk of liver cancer.

Depending on what kind of hepatitis a person has, there may be medicines to help fight it. Sometimes patients need to spend some days or weeks in a hospital if they feel too sick to eat and drink. Many people with hepatitis B feel better within six months.

PNEUMONIA

Pneumonia is an infection of the lungs and can be caused by a virus or bacteria. Early symptoms can include fever, chest pain, and vomiting. Pneumonia caused by bacterial infection will more likely lead to a sudden high fever and difficulty breathing. Pneumonia caused by a virus can be less severe.

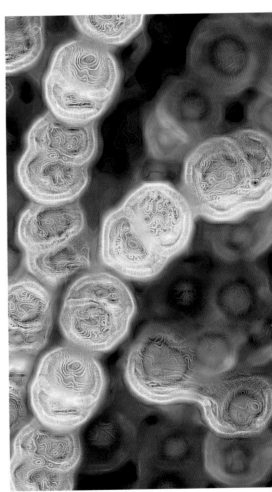

Doctors use physical exams, chest X-rays, and blood tests to diagnose pneumonia. All patients with pneumonia will be advised to get a lot of rest and drink plenty of fluids. Some kinds of pneumonia can also be treated with antibiotics. Very young children, or people over sixty-five years old, may need to be hospitalized when they

The streptococcus bacteria can cause pneumonia.

have pneumonia. In some cases, if the doctors believe the patient also has a virus, antiviral medications may be used to help combat the infection.

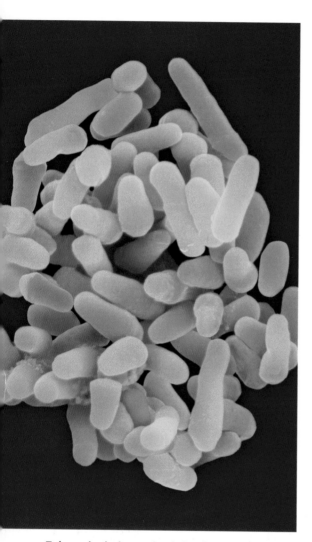

Tuberculosis bacteria thrive in cities with poor sanitation.

TUBERCULOSIS

Tuberculosis, commonly known as TB, is a disease caused by bacteria mainly affecting the lungs. It is a highly contagious illness that killed a large number of people in the 19th and early 20th centuries. Improved sanitation in cities and the development of a vaccine helped make TB rare in most of the world during the mid and late 20th century. Unfortunately, TB still exists in some parts of the world. One kind of TB that involves a serious fever that occurs over an extended period of time is called reactivation tuberculosis. This is a version of the illness in which the bacteria are not presently active, but can become active again at a later time. When the illness recurs, the patient will have a fever for a long period of time. If the disease progresses, the patient may begin coughing up blood. Tuberculosis can be prevented, and treated with medication, but if left untreated can be fatal.

MENINGITIS

Meningitis is a swelling of the tissue that covers the brain and spinal cord. Usually, it is caused by a bacterial or viral infection that comes from some other part of the body and spreads to the brain or spinal cord. Sometimes, something such as a serious ear infection or nasal sinus infection can lead to meningitis. Common symptoms include fever, irritability, a stiff neck, and lack of energy. Bacterial meningitis can be much more damaging to the nervous system than viral meningitis. If left untreated it can lead to hearing and eyesight problems, seizures, learning disabilities, or death.

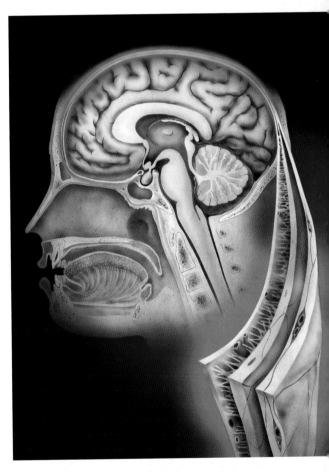

This illustration shows the cross-section of a human head. The meninges are three layers of tissue that protect the brain and spinal cord.

Fortunately, bacterial meningitis can be treated with antibiotics that are put directly into a person's veins. These treatments are done in a hospital over a few weeks. If the meningitis is caused by a virus, the doctor will advise the patient to rest and to take medication to help relieve headaches and body aches.

Q FEVER

Q fever is a disease caused by bacteria. Only half of all people with Q fever show symptoms; the rest may not even know they have the illness. Q fever can begin with a high fever (up to 104 to 105 °F or 40 to 40.6 °C) that may last as long as one to two weeks. Other symptoms include a severe headache, general fatigue and discomfort, joint pain, sore throat, confusion, nausea, vomiting, diarrhea, abdominal pain, and chest pain. One-third to one-half of the people who develop symptoms of Q fever will end up with pneumonia. And some patients with previous liver problems will develop a form of hepatitis. Q fever can be treated with antibiotics. The majority of people with Q fever will recover within a few months. In rare cases, however, it can be fatal.

RELAPSING FEVER

Some of the most dangerous illnesses that involve fever are characterized by a fever that recurs many times over a period of days or weeks. The term **relapsing fever** means that a fever will actually subside, and then return over and over again, multiple times. Malaria, blackwater fever, Colorado tick fever, rat-bite fever, dengue fever, and a large group of illnesses called African hemorrhagic fevers, all have relapsing fever as a main symptom.

MALARIA

Malaria is a common infectious disease in tropical climates that is caused by an organism called *Plasmodium*. Plasmodium is a parasite that is carried by mosquitoes. (Parasites are any animal, insect, or plant that lives off another **host** animal, insect, or plant, and causes it harm or does not benefit the host.) When a mosquito bites a human who has malaria, the mosquito becomes infected with the illness. Then, when the infected mosquito bites another human being, the Plasmodium parasite is transferred into the next person. Once inside the human, the parasite begins to multiply. Hundreds

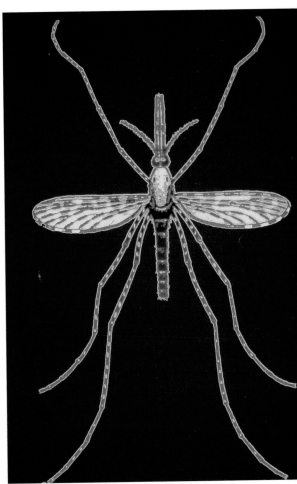

Malaria is carried by mosquitos infected with a parasite called Plasmodium.

of millions of people around the world are infected with malaria each year, but the disease is not common in the United States. Early symptoms of malaria can include trouble sleeping, lack of appetite, and irritability. Someone with malaria will usually then have chills followed by fever. In some cases, the fever may rise very suddenly to around 104 °F (40 °C) or higher. When the fever ends, the person will sweat intensely. And then the cycle will begin again. The patient may go through chills, fever, and sweating several times over a number of days.

People can protect themselves from malaria by sleeping under mosquito netting that is treated with insecticide. The illness can be cured with particular medicines. Unfortunately, these medicines are expensive for impoverished people around the world. If left untreated, malaria can be fatal.

BLACKWATER FEVER

Blackwater fever is a rare but serious illness. It is considered a very dangerous complication, or side effect, of a bad case of malaria. People who get blackwater fever most often have been infected by the parasite *Plasmodium falciparu*, and have had at least four attacks of malaria. A person with blackwater fever will have a high fever, chills, and a fast heartbeat. He or she will also produce urine that is dark red or black. The urine is this strange color because the parasite is destroying red blood cells and the body is releasing the dead cells through the urine.

Nets and Repellent

Because a mosquito can spread viruses from one infected person to other healthy people, it is important to keep a person with malaria, dengue fever, and other diseases isolated from any mosquitoes that might bite them and then transmit the disease to someone else. The easiest way to do this is with mosquito nets, window screens, and mosquito repellent.

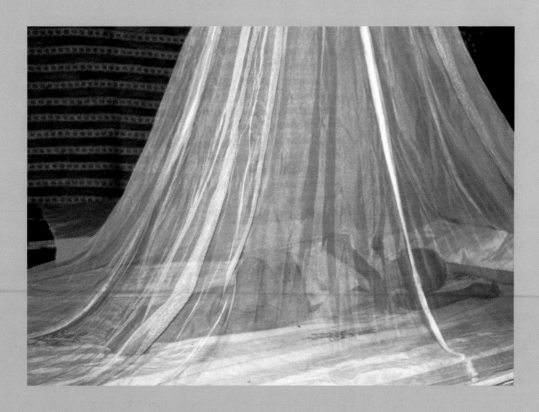

The illness is named for this symptom of dark urine. Because the parasite destroys so many red blood cells, the patient may very quickly become anemic, a condition in which one lacks red blood cells. Blackwater fever can be treated with whole-body blood transfusions and rest, but 25 to 50 percent of people with the illness will die from it.

COLORADO TICK FEVER (ALSO KNOWN AS MOUNTAIN FEVER)

Colorado tick fever is a virus that is passed to humans by the bite of a tick, called the *Dermacentor andersoni* tick, found mostly in the western regions of the United States. The state of Colorado is one area that is known for having many of these ticks. The virus actually lives for part of its life in a **mammal** (or warm-blooded animal with a spine) before it moves to the tick. The main animal that is known to carry the virus is the golden-mantled ground squirrel. Both the squirrels and the ticks are asymptomatic carriers. Only people bitten by the tick will suffer from the infection.

People are most likely to get sick with Colorado tick fever in the late spring and summer. Usually a few days after being bitten by an infected tick, a person will suddenly come down with a fever. He or she will feel achy in muscles and joints, and may have a headache, feel weak, and vomit. These symptoms may last two days. Then, after the symptoms disappear, they often will come back. A person with Colorado tick fever will sometimes feel much worse the second time around.

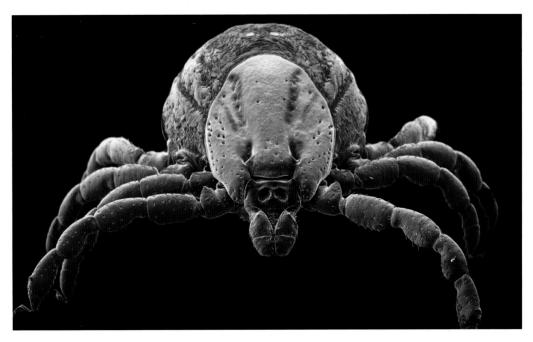

A close-up of *Dermacentor andersoni*, the tick that causes Colorado tick fever.

But once the patient finally recovers, he or she will never have Colorado tick fever again. The person will be **immune**.

There is no specific treatment for Colorado tick fever. Patients may take painkillers to relieve fever and pain.

RAT-BITE FEVER

Rat-bite fever, also known as sodoku, was first noticed in Japan. It is a bacterial infection that is transmitted through the bite of an infected rat. The incubation period of this disease can be anywhere from one week to one month. Five to twenty-eight days after an infected rat bites a person, he or she will suddenly see and feel symptoms. The bitten area will become swollen and hard, and the infected person will develop a fever. Both the pain of the swollen bite and the fever may come and go. The fever, and other symptoms, can disappear for several days and then reappear. Rat-bite fever can be treated with antibiotics. If it is left untreated, it can be fatal.

DENGUE FEVER

Dengue fever, also known as breakbone fever because of the pain it causes in joints, is a virus that is transmitted from one person to another by a mosquito. A mosquito can become infected with the virus by biting a person with dengue fever. Then, after eight to eleven days of incubation, if the mosquito bites someone else, the mosquito will transfer the virus into the new person. The main symptoms of dengue fever are a sudden, moderately high fever, severe pain in the joints, and intense pain behind the eyes.

A person infected with dengue fever is likely to experience nausea, vomiting, and loss of appetite. The fever will probably **subside**, or go down, for a little while and then return. The person will also get a rash within three to four days of getting the fever.

There is no treatment for dengue fever and it usually takes five to seven days for the fever to pass. Most people will recover fully. Some people, however, may develop a much more serious version of the disease called Dengue hemorrhagic fever. To **hemorrhage** means to bleed uncontrollably. When a person

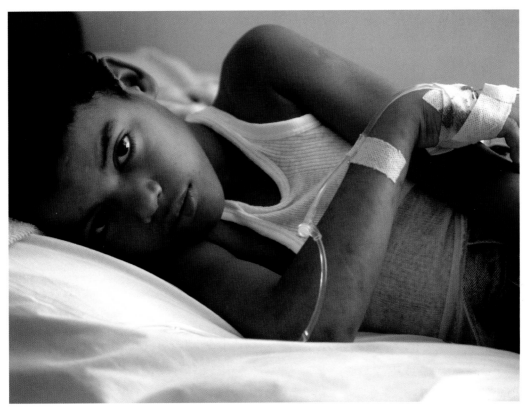

A young boy in the Dominican Republic suffering from Dengue fever.

has a hemorrhagic fever, he or she will bleed internally, and sometimes also externally. This can be very serious, and in some cases will lead to death.

There are four different **strains**, or kinds, of dengue fever. Once a person has had one kind of dengue fever, however, he or she becomes immune to it and cannot get that kind again. But he or she could still get one of the other strains. Dengue fever exists today primarily in Asia, but has also spread to parts of South America and Central America in recent decades.

Animals Can Get Fevers Too

African swine fever, also known as warthog fever, and hog cholera, also known as classical swine fever, are two dangerous diseases that infect pigs, hogs, wild boar, and other swine. In both cases, an infected animal will come down with a high fever. Once the fever has subsided, an animal with **acute** warthog fever is likely to die within two to seven days. An animal with hog cholera is more likely to die within seven days of the fever subsiding. There is no cure for either of these diseases but there is a vaccine to help prevent hog cholera.

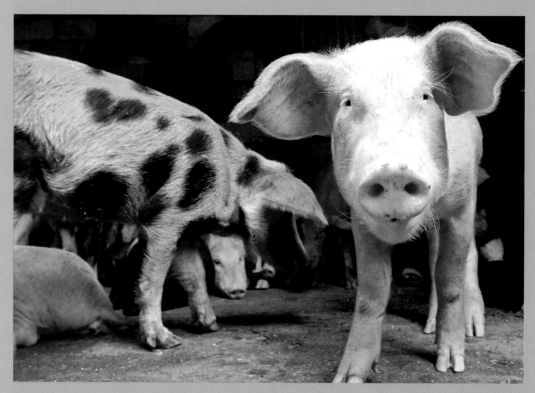

These pigs, at a farm in Nicaragua, were vaccinated in order to avoid getting swine fever.

VIRAL HEMORRHAGIC FEVERS (ALSO KNOWN AS AFRICAN HEMORRHAGIC FEVERS)

The term hemorrhagic fever refers to any one of a large group of illnesses that begin with a sudden fever, muscle and joint pain, and internal or external bleeding. The fever that marks the beginning of these viruses can last for the entire length of the illness, or it can come and go. These illnesses are known to cause liver damage and, in some cases, organ failure. Patients may go into shock from the sudden loss of blood or from organ failure.

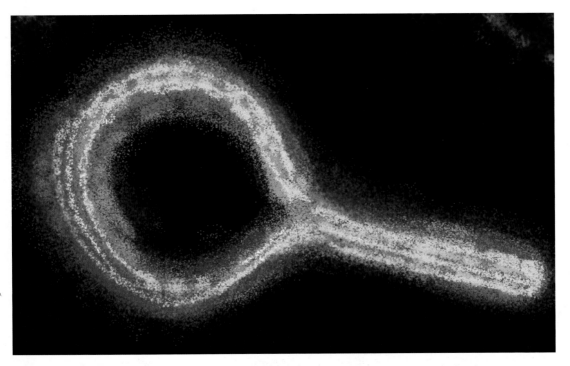

One of the most dangerous African hemorrhagic fevers is caused by the Ebola virus.

The viruses that cause hemorrhagic fevers are transmitted to people by ticks, mosquitoes, rats, or other insects and rodents. A person who has been infected will usually show symptoms, including fever, anytime from a few days to a few weeks from the time they were infected. There is no cure for viral hemorrhagic fevers. Treatment usually includes replacement of lost blood and fluids, and making the patient as comfortable as possible.

It is believed that hemorrhagic fevers have been around for centuries. Unfortunately, newer strains of viral hemorrhagic fevers have emerged in recent decades. Two of the most dangerous African hemorrhagic fevers are called the Ebola and Marburg viruses, and both are relatively new diseases that have very high fatality rates. Since Ebola was discovered in the 1970s there have been only four large outbreaks of the disease, but more than half of the people who contracted the disease died from it.

The Marburg virus was discovered in the late 1960s. Only a few people had contracted the disease until 1998, when there was a large outbreak of the disease in the Democratic Republic of the Congo. In 2004, there was another outbreak in Angola. In both cases, over 80 percent of the people who contracted the Marburg virus died from it.

Scientists do not know what animals or insects are carrying Ebola and Marburg, but they suspect that it may be bats.

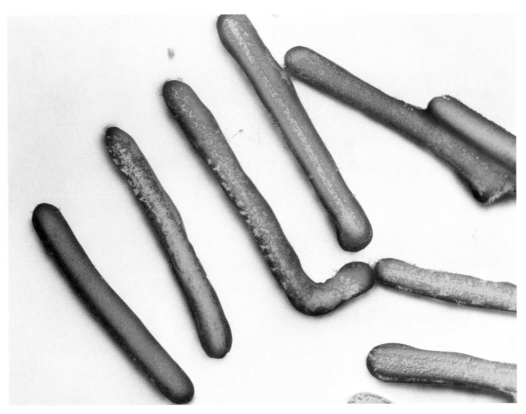

The Marburg virus causes a severe type of hemorrhagic fever that is often fatal.

Because scientists do not know what animals carry these illnesses, they do not know why outbreaks have occurred in specific places. It is known, however, that viral hemorrhagic fevers can spread from one infected person to another person through contact with infected blood or body fluids, such as saliva. This means that once a person has one of these viral hemorrhagic fevers, it can quickly spread from that person to others, and ultimately to a very large number of people.

3

THE HISTORY OF FEVER

Scientists do not know when humans started having fevers, but it is likely that human beings have had fevers throughout history. The word fever comes from the Latin word *febris*, which was related to a word that meant to warm, or heat.

For many centuries people believed that fever was an illness itself. They did not understand that fever is actually a symptom of illness. But since many people probably died of illness soon after getting a fever, it makes sense that people then thought fever was the illness.

With the invention of **thermometers** to measure fevers and medicines to treat

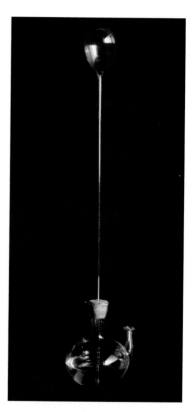

This thermoscope was built in the 1800s. The design was based on some of the same ideas Galileo used for his thermoscope in the 1500s.

illnesses involving fever, and other medical discoveries, people have been able to better understand the role of fever in illness.

THERMOMETERS

Any device used to measure temperature is called a thermometer. The word thermometer comes from two Greek words: *thermo* means heat and *meter* means to measure. Historians believe that an Italian scientist named Galileo Galilei invented the first thermometer in the late 1500s and called it a **thermoscope**. Galileo discovered that liquids expand when they get

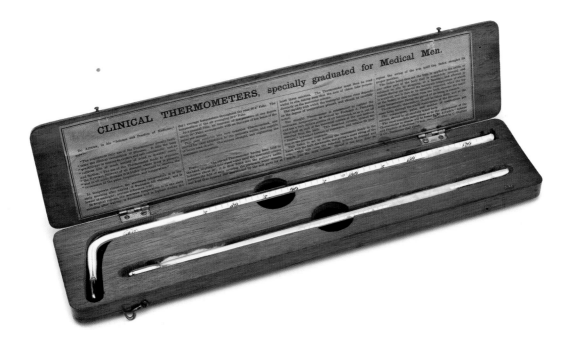

Thermometers were first used for medical purposes in the early 1600s. They were called clinical thermometers. Eventually they looked like this.

hotter, and contract when they get cooler. He made his thermoscope based on those discoveries.

In the years following Galileo's invention of the thermoscope, other scientists studied the properties of different liquids and were able to improve on the thermoscope. In addition, they focused on what kind of **temperature scale**, or units of measurement, to use to measure changes in temperature. An Italian doctor named Santorio, who lived in the same time period as Galileo, was the first person to put a numerical scale on the thermoscope. He was also the first to use a thermometer for medical purposes, and is credited with inventing the **clinical** thermometer in 1612.

The thermometers that we have today work differently from the thermoscope invented by Galileo, but many thermometers still rely on the basic idea that liquids expand and contract according to the temperature. Today we do use several types of temperature scales that were invented in the 1700s and 1800s. The two most widely used temperature scales are Fahrenheit and Celsius. Each is named for the scientist who invented it.

THERMOMETERS TODAY

For many years, a glass thermometer using mercury was the standard thermometer that almost every family owned. Today, there are many different kinds of thermometers that people can use at home. (In fact, thermometers with mercury are no longer

Fahrenheit Temperature Scale

A German scientist named Gabriel Daniel Fahrenheit developed the Fahrenheit temperature scale in the early 1700s. The Fahrenheit scale uses 32 degrees as the freezing point of water, 98.6 degrees for average body temperature, and 212 degrees as the boiling point of water. Each unit of the Fahrenheit scale is 1/180 of the difference between the freezing point and boiling points of water.

Celsius Temperature Scale

In 1742, a Swedish astronomer named Anders Celsius developed a temperature scale based on a total of 100 degrees. This scale was referred to as centigrade. *Centi* refers to 100, and *grade* is from the Latin meaning step. When Celsius first created the scale he used 0 degrees as the boiling point of water, and 100 degrees as the freezing point of water. Later these numbers were flipped. Zero degrees became the cold end of the scale, and 100 degrees was the hot end. The centigrade scale was renamed for its inventor in 1948. The Celsius temperature scale is still widely used around the world.

The mercury-in-glass thermometer was one of the first to use the Celsius scale of heat measurement.

recommended, because mercury is known to have some dangerous side effects—and glass thermometers can break.)

DIGITAL THERMOMETER

The most popular thermometer used in homes in the United States today is the digital thermometer. They come in many sizes and prices, and are readily available at pharmacies and supermarkets. Digital thermometers give quick and accurate temperature readings, and they can be used to take a temperature orally (in the mouth), rectally (in the bottom), or under the arm. The most accurate temperature reading is by taking it rectally. Using a thermometer orally and under the arm can produce reliable temperatures, too.

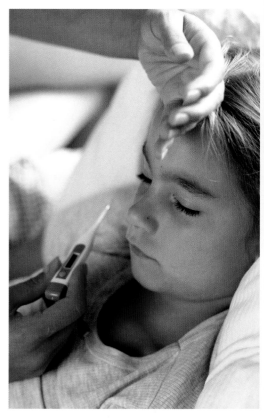

Digital thermometers are a quick and reliable way to get a body temperature reading.

ELECTRONIC EAR THERMOMETER

Another popular thermometer today is an electronic ear thermometer. These are the types most often used at the doctor's office. The doctor or nurse puts the probe

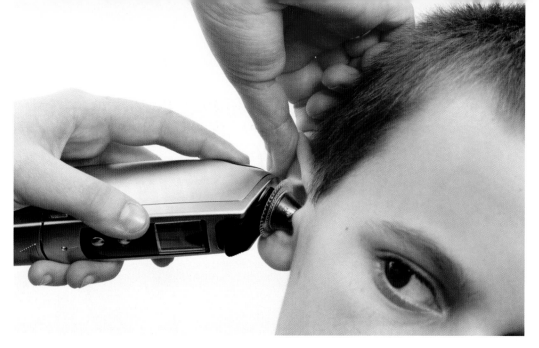

An ear thermometer is a more accurate way of getting a temperature reading and is usually used at doctors' offices and hospitals.

into a person's ear and takes the temperature inside the ear canal. These thermometers are quick and accurate but are not recommended for babies under three months old. Also, they can be expensive.

OTHER THERMOMETERS

Some other kinds of thermometers that are available today are not as reliable as digital or ear thermometers. Plastic-strip thermometers are small plastic strips that can be pressed against the forehead to see if someone has a fever. They were invented as an easy way to get a child's temperature, but they do not provide a reliable measure of an exact temperature. Pacifier thermometers were also invented to get an easy

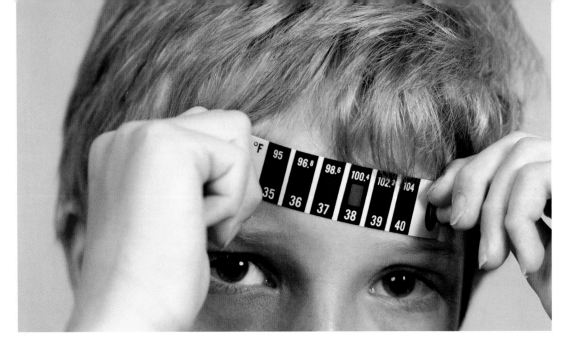

Another easy way to gauge body temperature is by using a plastic strip thermometer.

temperature reading on a young child. But like a regular oral thermometer, they need to stay in place for a few minutes, and that can be very difficult with young children.

TYPHOID: A HISTORIC FEVER

Throughout modern history, there have been numerous illnesses named for their fever symptoms. One of the most infamous historic illnesses involving fever that is still present today is typhoid fever.

Typhoid fever is a bacterial infection that usually enters the body when someone eats or drinks contaminated food or water. It can be spread among many people very quickly. This rapid spread of a disease is called an **epidemic**. There have been epidemics of typhoid fever around the world at various times throughout modern history. The disease is most often caused by pollution in a public water supply. Anywhere there is poor **sanitation**, local water can become infected by human or animal waste. Once someone has had typhoid fever, he or she can still carry the bacteria and infect other people, especially if the person does not wash his or her hands after using the bathroom and then handles food for others to eat. Polluted water and person-to-person transmission of the disease are just two of the ways an outbreak of typhoid fever can become an epidemic so rapidly.

ONE VERY LONG FEVER

One to three weeks after infection, a person with typhoid will have a headache and fever, feel achy, and may not be able to sleep. The fever will continue to rise over seven to ten days, until it peaks at 103 or 104 °F (39.4 to 40 °C). The fever can then last another ten days, or more, after reaching its peak. A person with typhoid can have the fever for a total of two to three or even four weeks! If the fever continues, other symptoms will usually become more intense as well. A patient may become delirious or confused. Once the fever begins to subside, other symptoms will also lessen. Today typhoid can be treated with antibiotics. If typhoid is left untreated, as many as 25 percent of those cases will end in death.

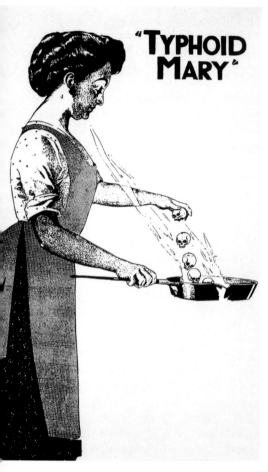

This cartoon shows typhoid Mary infecting the food she is cooking with deadly typhoid bacteria.

TYPHOID MARY

One of the most famous outbreaks of typhoid fever occurred in the New York area of the United States in the early 1900s. A woman named Mary Mallon was working as a cook in Oyster Bay, Long Island, when a number of people in the community came down with typhoid fever. It was recognized that she was carrying the typhoid bacteria, although she claimed she had never had typhoid herself. Although Mary promised not to work as a cook again, authorities traced several later outbreaks of typhoid back to her when it was discovered that she was moving from place to place and still working as a cook. In the end, more than fifty people became infected and three people were shown to have died from the typhoid they caught from Typhoid Mary. Many more are thought to have caught the disease from her, but it was never proven that their illnesses came from her. After being caught several times, Mary was committed to an isolation center for the rest of her life.

Typhoid Mary is not the only person to have spread the

illness to others over many years. Approximately 30 percent of people who have recovered from typhoid are considered transient carriers of the bacteria, which means that for some short period of time they can pass the illness to others. Approximately 5 percent of people who recover from typhoid will be long-term carriers, which means they can pass the illness to others for many, many years. It is likely that Mary Mallon may have had a mild case of typhoid earlier in her life and not realized it, or that she was an asymptomatic carrier. We will never know. But, to this day, a person carrying residual typhoid bacteria can give the illness to others if he or she does not wash frequently and/or wear gloves when handling food. This is why, even in cities with excellent sanitation, typhoid can reappear if someone who has been ill in the past is working in a restaurant, coffee shop, soup kitchen, or school cafeteria. Fortunately, government health officials do an excellent job of tracking cases of typhoid and making sure that people who carry the illness do not work with food.

Knowing that fever is a symptom of many illnesses, we understand that it can mark the beginning of either a serious illness or one that will pass easily within a short time. The development of modern thermometers has allowed people to keep track of fevers easily at home. Modern painkillers can help anyone with a fever feel more comfortable. A result of all of these modern innovations is that having a fever today is less stressful, and less risky, than it was in the past.

4

TREATING AND COPING WITH A FEVER

Having a fever is not any fun. It is uncomfortable and usually is accompanied by other symptoms. The good news is that most often a fever is something that will pass within a few hours or days. How a fever should be treated depends on the underlying cause of the fever. If the fever is the beginning of a cold or flu, no treatment may be needed. But if the fever is a symptom of pneumonia, or some other more serious illness, then treatment of the illness as well as the fever may be necessary.

When someone has a fever, the first thing to do is to take his or her temperature. Before taking a person's temperature, it is important to make sure that he or she has not had anything to eat or drink for twenty or thirty minutes, and that they have not just taken a bath or been very heavily bundled up. Eating and drinking can affect the temperature in the mouth. And taking a bath or being bundled up can also affect body temperature.

In order to get an accurate reading orally, the patient needs

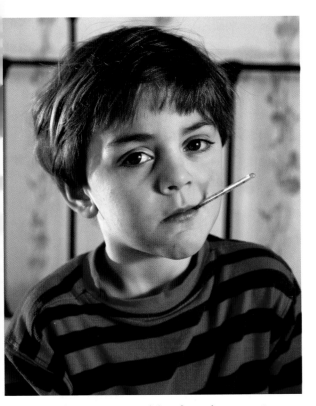

When a person with a fever has symptoms such as a rash, vomiting, or diarrhea, they should visit a doctor.

to keep the thermometer securely under the tongue for several minutes. If the patient is coughing, and cold air flows across the thermometer while it is in the mouth, the temperature reading will not be accurate. This is why children have their temperatures taken rectally, so that the doctor or caretaker taking the child's temperature can make sure the thermometer stays in place.

Temperature readings taken under the arm are considered accurate but they tend to read slightly lower than the temperature reading rectally. In general, 100.4 °F (38 °C) measured rectally is considered a fever. The equivalent temperature measured orally would be 99.5 °F (37.5 °C), and 99 °F (37.2 °C) if measured under the arm.

Once the temperature is determined, an adult can decide what to do next. If an adult has a fever below 102 °F (38.9 °C) and does not have any other symptoms, then it is probably safe for that person to take it easy and see what happens next. If a

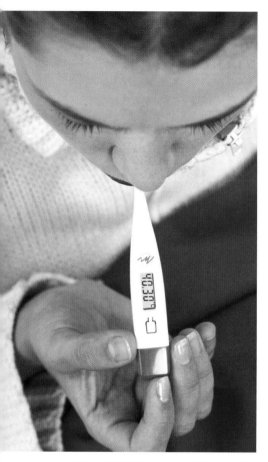

A reading of 99.5 degrees Fahrenheit, or 37.5 degrees Celsius, or higher, is considered a fever.

child has a fever below 102 °F (38.9 °C), a parent or other adult should get the child to rest, and watch for other symptoms. (The exception to this is newborns and infants under three months old, who should be taken to a doctor for any fever over 100.4 °F (38 °C).)

HOME TREATMENT

Bed rest and lots of fluids are the recommended home treatment for most mild to moderate fevers. Medication is not always recommended. Since the higher body temperature is helping to fight off infection, it can be good to let the fever run its course without taking medicine. Depending on whether the patient is shivering or sweating, he or she may want to wear warmer or cooler clothes. Taking a cool bath is also a simple and effective way to make someone with a fever more comfortable. If a person is, however, very uncomfortable, there are over-the-counter medications that can be used to bring the body temperature down.

Two medications that can help lower fever are acetaminophen

or ibuprofen. These medicines can lower a fever by blocking the pyrogens that tell the hypothalamus to make the body warmer. People used to take aspirin for a fever. But now we know that aspirin should not be given to children at any time, because it can cause a rare but dangerous illness called Reye's syndrome.

Perhaps most importantly, someone at home with a fever must be sure to drink plenty of water and other fluids. Even if the patient is not hungry or thirsty, it is very important to take in fluids in order to keep the body **hydrated**. When a person does not have enough water in his or her body, that person is **dehydrated**. Getting dehydrated is easy to do when a person's body

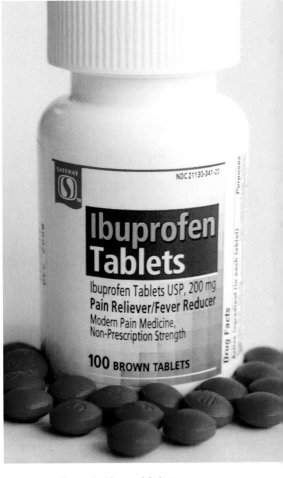

One way of combating a high temperature is to take ibuprofen, which is a medicine that helps to lower fever.

heats up with a fever. Being dehydrated is even more uncomfortable than having a fever, and can lead to other problems.

Here are some basic rules for deciding if a child with a fever must see a doctor. If the child is under three months old and has a fever, he or she should be taken to a doctor. If a child who is older than three months of age has a fever under 102 °F (38.9 °C), he or she probably does not have a serious illness if he or she still:

- is cheerful
- is playful
- is eating and drinking
- does not look seriously ill

A child does, however, need to see a doctor if he or she:

- has diarrhea or vomiting
- is dehydrated, and/or will not drink
- complains of an earache, sore throat, or specific pain
- still has a fever after one day—when he or she is younger than two years old
- still has a fever after three days—when he or she is three years old or older
- has fevers repeatedly for a few hours over several nights

For an adult, the rules are basically the same. If an adult has a fever under 102 °F (38.9 °C) and is generally feeling well and interested in eating and drinking, then a doctor is not necessary. That adult should see a doctor, however, if he or she begins vomiting or does not want to drink, complains of discomfort, or has the fever for a few days.

VISITING A HEALTH CARE PROVIDER

If a fever is accompanied by other symptoms, such as a rash, vomiting, or diarrhea, the ill person should see a doctor as soon as possible. Once the doctor diagnoses the underlying illness, he or she will be able to treat the patient's illness and fever. In many cases, the fever will have already passed by the time a patient gets to a doctor. If the patient has a bacterial infection, such as pneumonia or strep throat, the doctor will probably prescribe antibiotics. If, however, it is a type of viral infection, such as the flu, the doctor will probably advise bed rest and drinking a lot of liquid. If

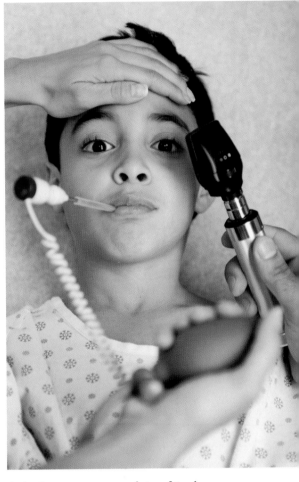

A doctor may use a variety of tools to examine a patient, and diagnose their illness.

the fever persists and is making the patient very uncomfortable, over-the-counter medications can be given to lower the fever. These are the same medications that would be given at home, including acetaminophen or ibuprofen.

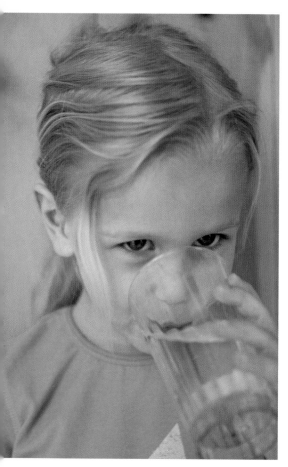

Anyone with a fever should drink fluids to stay hydrated.

SIDE EFFECTS OF FEVER

Most fevers go away in a relatively short time and have few side effects. But with a very high, long-lasting fever, or a fever in conjunction with other symptoms, watch for side effects. The most dangerous potential side effect of fever is dehydration. After a fever has served its purpose, the body will begin to sweat. The sweat running over the outside of the skin will bring the temperature of the skin and the entire body down. During this process, however, the body is losing valuable fluids. Drinking plenty of clear liquids is the best way to ensure that a person will maintain a good fluid balance during an illness. One way to be sure someone has been drinking enough fluid is to keep track of how often he or she urinates. If someone does not urinate for a very long period of time, it is likely that he or she is dehydrated. Another sign of dehydration is when someone really does not want to drink, or says that water makes him or her nauseous.

Other side effects of serious fever can include irritability, confusion, hallucinations, and convulsions. Very young children sometimes will have a seizure in reaction to a fever. This is relatively rare and usually harmless, but is a very scary experience for parents. Children who are prone to **febrile** seizures will usually outgrow them by the time they are five to six years old.

PREVENTING FEVER

There is no guaranteed way to prevent a fever. The only thing a person can do to avoid fever is to avoid being exposed to infectious diseases. The most effective way to do that is to wash one's hands a number of times throughout the day. It is important to wash hands with soap and warm water, and it is a good idea to do it just before eating and right after using the toilet. Basically, anytime a person has been in contact with germs from an animal or another person, it is a good idea to wash up. Also, if someone who is sick touches another person's hand, or hands someone else a pencil, it is important that the healthy person does not then touch his or her own mouth or eyes until after washing. This kind of casual contact is the way most viral infections are passed from person to person.

No one enjoys having a fever. But it can be reassuring to know that many fevers are just the first sign of a common cold or flu. While someone might be upset at the idea of being sick,

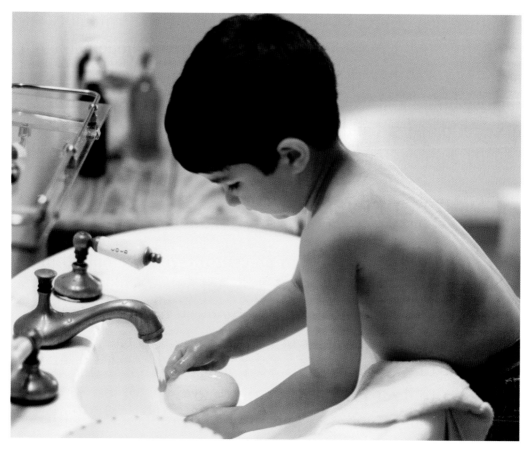

Washing your hands with soap and water is one of the most effective ways to avoid getting sick with a fever.

it is important to remember that fever is actually one way that the body combats illness. If the fever is serious, it is very likely that a doctor can help. Doctors are very good at diagnosing illnesses, and today there are many effective treatments.

GLOSSARY

acute—A term used to describe a fever or illness that gets worse rapidly, and is severe.

asymptomatic carrier—A human, animal, or insect that has an illness but shows no symptoms or signs of the illness.

bacteria—Very small living cells that can only be seen using a microscope; some are beneficial to the body and others can cause illness or disease.

clinical—A tool or practice used in medical treatment.

contagious—Capable of being spread through contact, or being infected with a disease that can be spread.

dehydrated—The condition of having too little water and body fluids within the body.

diagnose—The process of identifying the cause of a problem or illness.

epidemic—A sudden, rapid outbreak of disease that spreads widely and effects many individuals at one time.

febrile—Feverish, caused by a fever.

fever—A higher than normal body temperature.

flu—An illness caused by a virus, also known as influenza.

germ—A term commonly used to describe bacteria, viruses, parasites, and other microorganisms that cause illness.

hemorrhage—To lose blood uncontrollably, often from a blood vessel.

host—The organism upon which a parasite lives.

hydrated—The condition of having sufficient water and body fluids within the body.

hypothalamus—The part of the brain that controls body temperature and other bodily functions.

illness—Sickness or disease.

immune—Resistant to a disease.

immune system—The bodily system that protects the body from foreign substances, cells, and infection by recognizing these foreign invaders and destroying them.

infection—An illness caused by bacteria, viruses, parasites, or other pathogens that the immune system has not yet destroyed.

leukocytes—White blood cells.

lymph nodes—The structures found throughout the immune system where white blood cells are located.

mammal—A warm-blooded animal with a spine.

parasite—Organisms that live in or on other living things, called hosts. Parasites often cause the host harm.

pathogens—Bacteria or viruses that can cause disease or illness.

pyrexia—Fever.

pyrogen—A chemical produced by the body that tricks the brain into thinking that the body is cooler than it is, in order to induce a fever and fight off a virus or bacteria.

relapsing fever—A term that describes illnesses in which fever will subside and return, over and over again.

saliva—Fluid produced by glands in the mouth to keep the mouth moist for speech and to help digest food.

sanitation—The process of killing or removing germs and waste.

strains—Related groups of viruses that have slightly different characteristics.

subside—To diminish, or pass.

symptom—Any change in the body that signals the presence of an illness.

temperature scale—Units of measurement used to indicate changes in temperature.

thermometer—A tool that measures change in temperature.

thermoscope—The first thermometer, invented by Galileo.

upper respiratory tract—The nose, throat, and trachea (or windpipe).

virus—A tiny living particle that can cause illness or disease.

FIND OUT MORE

Books

Isle, Mick. *Everything You Need to Know About Colds and Flu*. New York: Rosen Publishing, 2004.

Murphy, Jim. *An American Plague: The True and Terrifying Story of the Yellow Fever Epidemic of 1793*. New York: Clarion Books, 2003.

Web Sites

KidsHealth: A kid's guide to fever
http://www.kidshealth.org/kid/ill_injure/sick/fever.html

Mayo Clinic Tools for Healthier Lives
http://www.mayoclinic.com/health/fever/DS00077

PBS: The Most Dangerous Woman in America (Typhoid Mary)
http://www.pbs.org/wgbh/nova/typhoid/

INDEX

Page numbers for illustrations are in **boldface**

ABOUT THE AUTHOR

Camilla Calamandrei loves all kinds of nonfiction stories and believes that truth really *is* stranger than fiction. She has been a writer and editor of science and history books for young adults since 2004. She is also an award-winning documentary filmmaker and designer of interactive media for children.

CC

THOMAS CRANE PUBLIC LIBRARY

3 1641 0082 1582 8

Central Children's

JAN 2009